—— The Patient's Guide ——

MRI

ADAM E. M. ELTORAI
JIN JUNG
TERRANCE T. HEALEY

Praeclarus Press, LLC
©2019 Jin Jung. All rights reserved.

www.PraeclarusPress.com

Praeclarus Press, LLC
2504 Sweetgum Lane
Amarillo, Texas 79124 USA
806-367-9950
www.PraeclarusPress.com

DISCLAIMER
The information contained in this publication is advisory only and is not intended to replace sound clinical judgment or individualized patient care. The author disclaims all warranties, whether expressed or implied, including any warranty as the quality, accuracy, safety, or suitability of this information for any particular purpose.

ISBN: 978-1-946665-25-6

©2019 Jin Jung. All rights reserved.

Email: ejkjung424@gmail.com

Cover Design: Ken Tackett

Developmental Editing: Kathleen Kendall-Tackett

Copy Editing: Chris Tackett

Layout & Design: Nelly Murariu

CONTENTS

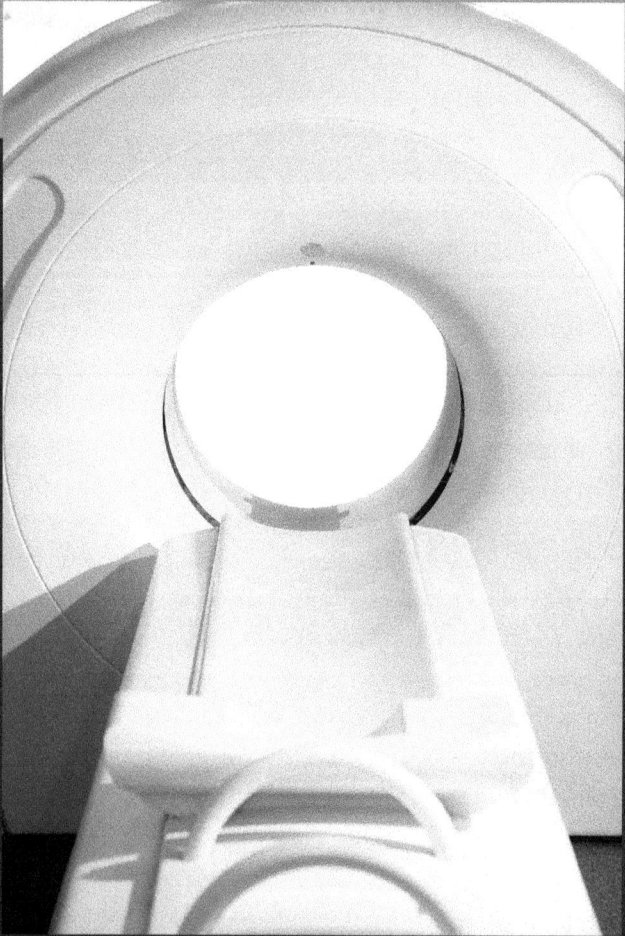

WHAT IS MRI?

MRI stands for Magnetic Resonance Imaging and was discovered by Sir Peter Mansfield and Paul C. Lauterbur. They were awarded the Nobel Prize in Medicine in 2003.

An MRI uses the strength of the magnetic field produced by an electric current and pulsed radio waves that result in images of organs and other structures inside your body. The detail of how MRI works to produce an image involves a lot of complex physics and is beyond the scope of this discussion.

Just know that the MRI unit creates a near uniform magnetic field, which acts on the hydrogen molecules in our body (present in water – 60% of the human body is made up of water).

We are able to record magnetic signals from the way these hydrogen molecules interact in our bodies in the MRI scanner through computer processing. The end result is MRI images that a board-certified radiologist interprets. The radiologist interprets the images, which helps doctors provide patients with appropriate treatment.

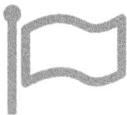

MRI is generally safe and painless.

Its exterior appearance may be similar to the CT scanner, but it does not expose the patient to ionizing radiation. Just as with CT, an MRI scan can be performed with or without contrast. Contrast is administered into blood vessels through a small IV (intravenous) line in the arm.

WHY IS IT PERFORMED?

MRI is another medical imaging tool (i.e., CT, ultrasound, and X-rays) that can be used to diagnose a wide variety of problems or abnormal conditions in different parts of the body. It provides different types of information to doctors about the body part compared to CT or ultrasound. Patients often ask why they need both a CT and an MRI. Specifically, MRI provides imaging with great contrast between different types of tissues within our body to allow identification of abnormal tissue.

Most commonly, it is used to image the brain, spine, liver, kidneys, adrenal glands, pancreas, prostate, breasts, heart, knee, shoulder, hip, and pelvis.

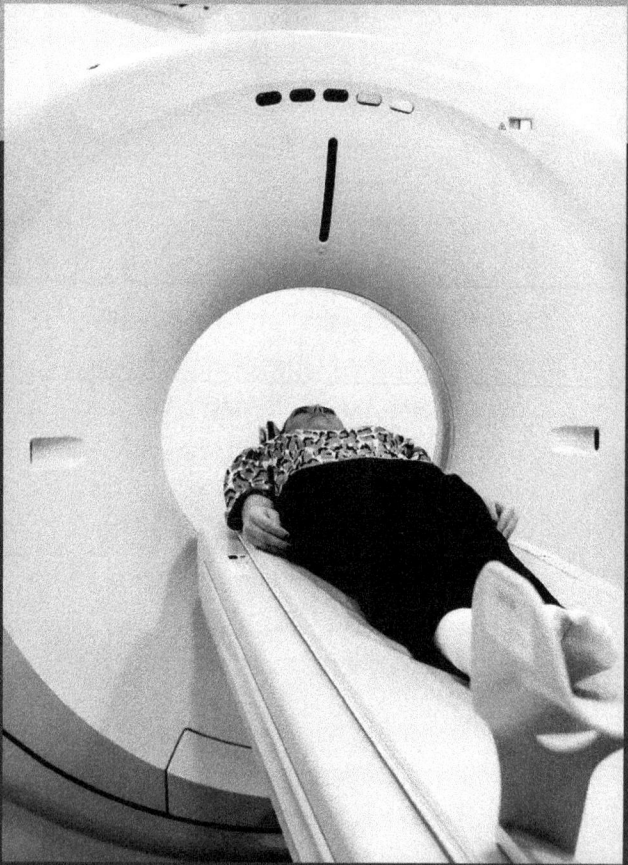

HOW DO I PREPARE?

Once your doctor has ordered an MRI to be performed, you will be asked many questions concerning your past medical conditions and procedures. In some cases, a patient's pre-existing condition may be a contraindication for an MRI to be performed. Usually, this check is performed briefly over the phone by the MRI scheduler prior to appointment date. A more thorough check is performed by a radiology staff member on the day of the appointment, prior to the examination.

One should communicate to the staff or technologist about any of the particular conditions below:

- Pacemaker or defibrillator

- Diabetes

- Pregnancy

- Spine stimulator/Neurostimulator

- Joint replacement

- Kidney disease/issues

- Heart valves

- Insulin pump or any implanted drug devices

- Aneurysm clips or coils

- Ear implants

- Tattoos or body piercings

- Anxiety or claustrophobia

- Exposure to metal or history of being metal worker

- Allergy to Gadolinium contrast

- Any other conditions you are concerned about, which may alter the MRI scan

Some of the above conditions can be worked around. For example, for claustrophobia or anxiety, your doctor can prescribe you with medications, which will allow you to be able tolerate the exam. Patients with other more complicated or non-compatible conditions may not be able to have an MRI scan.

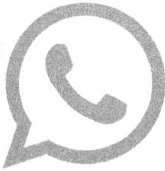

Make sure you doublecheck with your doctor or radiologist prior to the day of your MRI scan to ensure you do not need to drink or prep.

Usually, there are no limitations for eating and drinking on the day prior to the exam. In some cases, especially if you are having a MRI examination of your abdomen, you may be asked to fast for a short time interval. This is especially true if you are planning to undergo an examination called MR Enterography (MRE), where the goal is to examine your small bowel. However, you should doublecheck with you doctor or radiologist prior to the day of your MRI scan to ensure you do not need to drink or prep.

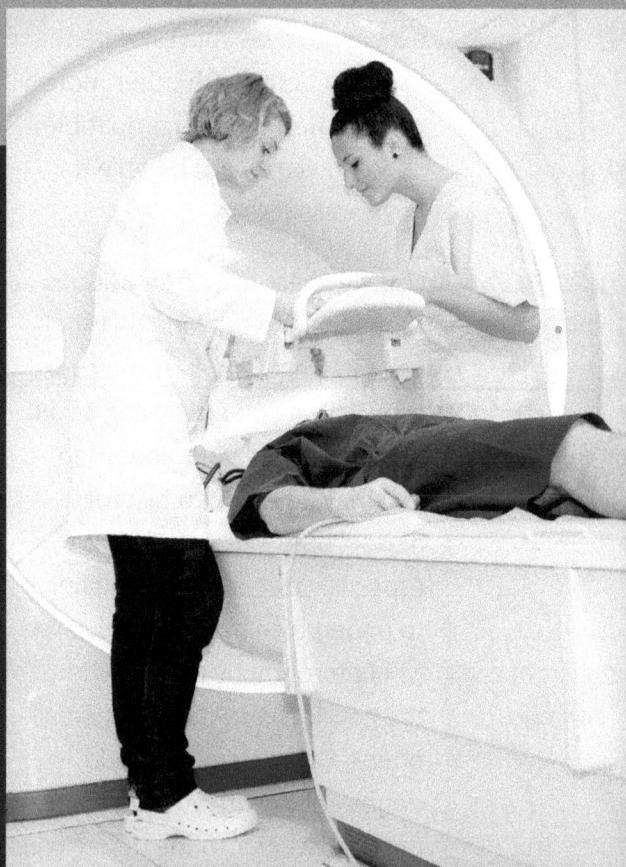

THE EQUIPMENT

The MRI equipment is made up of a large tube-like structure, which contains a large circular magnet with variable strength. This strength is measured in Tesla (T). Most common is the 1.5 T magnet. However, 3.0 T magnets are becoming more commonly available.

The center of the MRI has a bed for the patient to lie comfortably. Most MRI scanners are such that the patient will be surrounded within the center of the magnet during the length of the examination. Some centers are able to provide Open MRI, which does not surround the patient. This is sometimes used for patients who have severe anxiety or claustrophobia.

The drawback to these magnets are that they usually provide lower quality images due to low magnetic field strength capabilities, which may make it slightly more difficult for the radiologist interpreting the images. There are also extremity-based MRI units, which are available in select health care systems.

Smaller equipment involved in the MRI scan are coils, which send and receive radio waves. Some are within the MRI unit and are responsible for the loud noises during the exam. Other coils, such as the "head" or "body" coil, are closer to the body part being imaged to allow for higher quality images.

THE
PROCESS

The whole process starts off with you checking in at the front desk. Usually the office asks you arrive approximately 30 to 45 minutes prior to the examinations to allow adequate time for completing medical paperwork and an extensive pre-procedure check.

After checking in at the front desk, the MRI technologist asks about any potential conditions (discussed above) that may interfere with or prevent the MRI scan. Usually after this check, the patient is then directed to change into a hospital gown. If your doctor ordered the

MRI with contrast, a physician, nurse, or technologist will insert an intravenous (IV) line into a vein on your arm to inject contrast material at the time of the exam.

By now, you are in the room with the MRI scanner. You will be placed in the bed at the center of the magnet. Patients are usually provided earphones or headsets so that they can listen to music or audio of their choice during the exam (since it's loud). Don't be surprised when you hear loud, intermittent, banging noises in the scanner. It's all part of the unit working in sync.

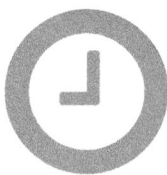

Most MRI exams last approximately 30 to 40 minutes

The exam time varies based on the body part being imaged and if you received contrast. Most exams last approximately 30 to 40 minutes.

MRI imaging centers clearly identify four zones you should be aware of.

ZONE 1

Public Zone. Safe from magnetic field and farthest from the MRI scanner (for example – front desk)

ZONE 2

Screening Zone. Outside the MRI scanner and control room (for example – patient change room)

ZONE 3

Last Zone closest to MRI scanner room. (Examples: MRI technologist in control room)

ZONE 4

Inside the room with the MRI scanner. Metals and unscreened pacemakers not allowed!

Also note that, unlike X-rays or CT (Computed Tomography) scans, the MRI exam does not expose you to ionizing radiation.

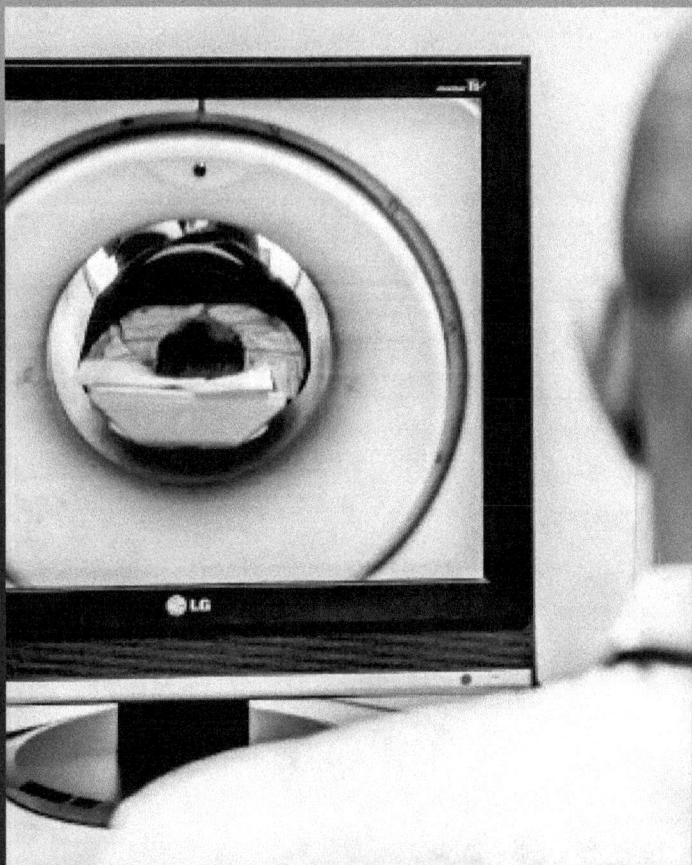

AFTER
THE PROCEDURE

After the procedure, the technologist will direct you back into the changing room. Once you've changed out of the gown, you are free to leave. Images are sent for the radiologist to interpret that day or the next day. Depending on examination and health care system, your results may reach your doctor within 1 to 2 days, but usually no longer than 5 to 7 days. You should check with your doctor's office if you are not notified of your results within 7 days.

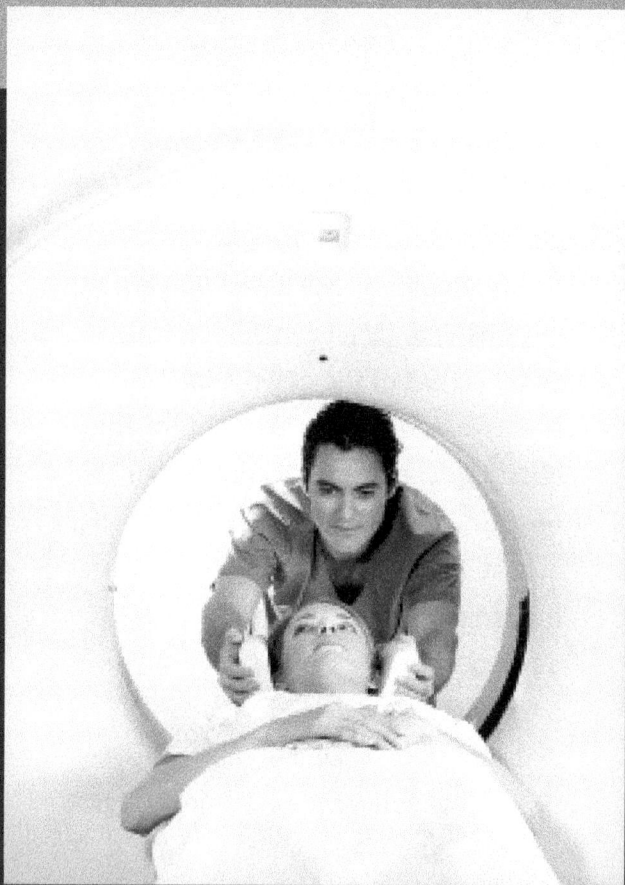

BENEFITS VS. RISKS OF MRI

B enefits of having an MRI is that it can be used to obtain information about the body part being imaged in order for your doctor to provide you with appropriate treatment for a possible abnormal condition. It is different from a CT scanner or X-ray in that it provides different types of information and produces no radiation exposure.

There are no known risks of having an MRI in the absence of pre-existing conditions described earlier. There are no known health hazards from exposure to a strong magnetic field, even in pregnancy. Most common complications/risks include skin burns in patients with tattoos, or skin-to-skin contact in the scanner, which are largely preventable by appropriate pre-scan measures.

The exception to absent risk is when contrast is given to the patient. The type of contrast, which is used for MRI exams, is gadolinium-based contrast agents (GBCAs). Unfortunately, not everything is known about the risks of gadolinium at this time. We do know that in some patients who receive frequent examinations with contrast that the gadolinium deposits in certain parts of the body. It is unknown whether deposits in the body lead to harmful effects.

There is a condition known as Nephrogenic Systemic Fibrosis (NSF), which is relevant only to patients with underlying kidney disease. Simply, it is a condition that causes abnormal skin changes. More information regarding this condition and treatment is being sought out as we speak. Just note that risks are **rare.**

LIMITATIONS

U sually, there are only two situations that limit MRI scans ability to provide an adequate image.

1. Metal in the body (for example, joint replacement, aneurysm coil, metal plate for fracture fixation, surgical clips).

2. Size of the patient
   a. Image quality may be negatively affected in obese patients, as this introduces increased background noise.

   b. Most commonly used MRI units have a maximum allowable diameter of 60 cm. If a patient's body diameter approaches or exceeds this measurement, patient may need to undergo scanning in an open MRI instead. This is due to concerns for heating, when the skin makes contact with the MRI unit.

c. Patients weighing greater than 325 lbs may not be able to undergo MRI scan in the commonly used scanners, although some units support up to 440 lbs. Make sure to check with the MRI technologist, if this pertains to you.

FREQUENTLY ASKED QUESTIONS

Is it painful?

No. The only exception is a patient with tattoos or body piercings, for which appropriate pre-MRI treatment should occur prior to imaging.

Does MRI cause radiation exposure?

No. MRI uses magnetic field and radio waves without use of ionizing radiation like CT or X-ray.

Is MRI harmful?

No. MRI in itself is not harmful.

When and why is contrast administered?

Gadolinium-based contrast is administered to accentuate the difference in tissue contrast and make tumors/cancers much more easily visible.

Is contrast harmful?

In patients with kidney disease, contrast can be harmful in certain conditions. You should check with your doctor and/ or radiologist prior to having contrast administered if you have kidney disease.

GLOSSARY

COIL

One of many components that make up the MRI. It is used to receive and send signals in order to make up an image.

COMPUTED TOMOGRAPHY (CT)

Commonly referred as "CAT scan." It is a medical-imaging tool, which uses a series of X-rays to produce an image of the body. It results in radiation exposure to the body.

CONTRAST

An agent given through an IV that increases the visibility of blood vessels and tumors/masses in our bodies.

ELECTRIC CURRENT

Simply refers to moving electric charge. In MRI, this is used to create a magnetic field.

GADOLINIUM-BASED CONTRAST AGENTS (GBCA)

Contrast agent used in MRI.

INTRAVENOUS (IV)

Refers to administration into a vein (type of blood vessel).

IONIZING RADIATION (RADIATION)

Energy carried by a particle or X-rays that has the ability to alter the tissues, which it passes through. It is used in medical imaging.

KIDNEY DISEASE

Abnormal condition of the kidney, which may be chronic or acute.

MAGNETIC FIELD

A nonvisible magnetic force, created by running electric current used in MRI scanners.

MAGNETIC RESONANCE IMAGING (MRI)

Simply refers to imaging resulting from manipulation of magnetic field and radio waves. There is no radiation exposure to the patient.

MAGNETIC RESONANCE ENTEROGRAPHY (MRE)

MRI used to examine the small bowel.

NEPHROGENIC SYSTEMIC FIBROSIS (NSF)

Rare condition that occurs in individuals with kidney disease who received GBCAs. The full extent of this condition is not currently well known. However, some of the described symptoms include abnormal skin changes. This is one of many reasons that patients with underlying kidney disease are strictly screened prior to receiving contrast.

NOISE

MRI signal that does not contribute to diagnostic medical imaging. This is increased in various conditions, especially in obesity.

SIGNAL

Refers to data provided to the computer from MRI unit. This allows us to create an image, which can be interpreted by a radiologist.

TISSUE CONTRAST

Refers to differences in appearance of nearby tissue in imaging.

ULTRASOUND (US)

Imaging tool that uses soundwaves. There is no radiation exposure to the patient.

X-RAYS (XR)

Man-made energy wave used in medicine to produce imaging. This exposes patients to radiation.

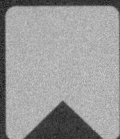

ADDITIONAL RESOURCES

www.radiologyinfo.org

www.fda.gov

www.acr.org

MY CONTACTS

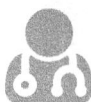

NAME

CONTACT

NAME

CONTACT

NAME

CONTACT

NAME

CONTACT

MY APPOINTMENTS

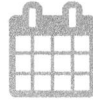

MONDAY
Date:
_____

THURSDAY
Date:
_____

TUESDAY
Date:
_____

FRIDAY
Date:
_____

WEDNESDAY
Date:
_____

SATURDAY
Date:
_____

MY QUESTIONS

MY QUESTIONS

MY NOTES

MY NOTES

MY NOTES

www.ingramcontent.com/pod-product-compliance
Lightning Source LLC
Chambersburg PA
CBHW060502210326
41520CB00015B/4056